Fat Burning F

An A-Z list of Foods that Burn Fat to Start a Healthy Diet

By C Elias

Introduction

Obesity is a worldwide crisis. Today, people all over the world struggle to control their weight. Many of these people want a quick fix to their problem. In order to quickly reduce their weight, many of these people have tried popular diets or weight loss supplements to lose the weight. While people may get the effect they want using these methods, they will quickly gain back their weight once they begin to eat "normally" again.

The average person eats a diet that consists of sugar, fat, and carbohydrates. This unhealthy diet also contributes to weight gain. The good news is that there is a better way to lose weight and stay healthy. One of the easiest and best ways to lose weight and keep that weight off is to include some of these fat fighting foods in your daily diet.

When you eat foods that help fight fat, it doesn't mean that these foods will offset your fat and calorie intake or that you won't store fat. It means that these foods can help to increase your metabolism. When your metabolism is functioning at peak efficiency, your body can easily break down fat and get rid of toxins in your body.

The concept is pretty simple actually. When you overeat or eat the wrong types of food, you will put on weight. Therefore, If you eat the right foods you should start to lose weight. This is especially true when you add fat burning foods into your diet.

The purpose of this book is to teach you about these fat fighting foods as well as explaining a little bit about how these foods can help you to lose weight.

Keep in mind that this list does not include an exhaustive list of the fat fighting foods found all over the world. The list still is pretty thorough and impressive though. It includes fruits and vegetables you have heard of and perhaps some you haven't.

If you really want to increase your weight loss, you may want to decrease your fat and sugar intake. This also can do wonders to improve your health. Just eating a lot of fat fighting foods will not help you to lose weight.

Remember that you need a varied diet to get all the vitamins and minerals that you need. Proper nutrition ensures that your body is working at peak efficiency. While eating cantaloupes for extended periods of time may help you to lose weight, it will certainly have a negative impact on your health and nutrition. A healthy menu will include fruits, vegetables, meat, and breads. Limiting the amount of sugar and fat in your diet will also help.

Diet is only half of the solution when you are trying to lose weight. In addition to improving your diet you will also need to exercise. Exercise will help your body to burn calories as well as fat. You do not have to join a gym or exercise for hours a day in order to improve your health. Even a simple exercise routine like walking around your neighborhood each day can help.

The thing that most diets don't tell you is that you will gain your lost weight back if you go back to an unhealthy lifestyle. This is why fad diets do not work. If you exercise regularly and gradually improve your diet, you can lose weight and keep it off. This e-book will help you to do just that.

C Elias
www.effective-diets.com

"A"

Apple

According to an old say, an apple helps to keep the doctor away. Apples also can help to increase you metabolism and help you to melt fat. Apples have contain pectin which helps you to feel full. If you feel full, chances are that you will eat less.

According to studies, pectin also can limit the amount of fat that can be absorbed by cells. Dieters who ate an apple before a meal lost about 1/3 more than the group that did not. Because apples are sweet, eating an apple can also help to cut down on your junk food consumption.

Apples are loaded with Vitamin C. This can help your immune system, but it can also help to break up fat so it can be flushed out of your system easier.

Artichokes

Artichokes contain a substance called Silymarin. In studies, it has been shown that this substance can help improve digestion. Silymarin also can help to detoxify your liver, lower blood sugar levels, and improve your cholesterol levels. This combination will help to improve your health as well as help you to lose weight.

This power packed vegetable is definitely worth a try. Pick up some artichokes on your next shopping trip and see for yourself!!

Asparagus

Asparagine is a chemical contained in Asparagus that helps improve kidney function as well as circulation. This chemical can also help to break down oxalic acid. This particular acid helps to bind fat to cells. By breaking up the oxalic acid, the asparagus can help to reduce your fat levels.

Apricots

Apricots are a wonderful food to eat. This fruit is high in fiber and can aid in proper digestion and help the digestive tract to function properly.

Fruits high in fiber tend to help decrease your appetite because they enable you to feel full. In addition, fiber can help to reduce your cholesterol levels which will improve your health.

Apricots also contain a high amount of beta-carotene which is an antioxidant. According to studies, antioxidants are helpful in that they help rid the body of dangerous toxins. People who incorporate beta-carotene into their diets can help to prevent cancer, cataracts, and even heart disease.

"B"

Beets

Beets are regarded as a natural diuretic. A diuretic will flush out fats and excess fluid from your body.

Beets also contain iron which can help to cleanse your red blood cells, making it more difficult for fat cells to deposit to them.

Beets also contain therapeutic amounts of naturally occurring chlorine. This natural chlorine also can help to clear toxins and fats from your body.

Finally, beets are high in fiber which mean that eating them will help your digestive system as well as your circulatory system.

Brussel Sprouts

Do you remember how your mother used to force you to eat brussel sprouts? It turns out that your mom was right; you should eat your brussel sprouts!

Brussel sprouts are good because they are high in protein and low in fat and calories. You could make a meal out of this vegetable just by adding grains.

Sprouts are also high in Vitamin C as well as fiber. This combination can help you to lose weight will allowing you to feel full.

Finally, brussel sprouts have been shown to reduce fat deposits around the stomach. This is because the spouts contain phytonutrients which can break down this type of specific fat deposits.

Eating sprouts can also help to jump start your metabolism and help you to burn calories more efficiently.

Broccoli

Broccoli is loaded with fiber. Broccoli also contains phytonutrients and is a great gut busting vegetable. By eating broccoli, you can help to decrease the amount of fat around your stomach.

Finally, broccoli has large quantities of Vitamin C which can help to dilute fat so it can easily be flushed from your system.

Blackberries

Blackberries also are packed with fiber. These tasty berries are great to eat by themselves or over a bowl of healthy cereal.

When you eat blackberries, you are also getting a large dose of Vitamin C. This vitamin can help your immune system and it can help your body to flush toxins and fat from your body.

Blackberries are called a miracle food because it actually takes more calories to digest these delicious berries that it does to eat them.

Keep these naturally sweet berries on hand for when you get a craving for something sweet!

Blueberries

Lately, blueberries have been referred to as a superfood. It is true that blueberries are a low calorie food that is high in vitamins.

Blueberries can also help to fight stomach fat and the berries are chock full of phytonutrients and antioxidants. Antioxidants can help to decrease your risks of developing cancer and other types of diseases.

Because blueberries are sweet, but are low in sugar, eating them is a great way to deal with sugar cravings. Instead of having a cookie, you may want to try a bowl full of blueberries instead.

Blueberries also freeze nicely. If you freeze some fresh blueberries during the summer time, you can enjoy the berries even when they aren't in season.

Beans

Beans are a wonderful protein source. In fact, a half a cup of cooked beans actually contains more protein than several ounces of meat!

In addition to being a great source of protein, beans also contain a large amount of fiber. Not only will this keep your digestive tract working properly, but it will also keep your stomach full.

If you like variety, you will especially love eating beans. There are a number of different types of beans including kidney beans, lima beans, pinto beans and navy beans.

"C"

Cabbage

Cabbage contains sulphur and iodine. While combining both of those ingredients in your body may sound unhealthy, there is nothing to worry about. In fact, the combination of the two helps to keep your stomach and intestines clean.

Cabbage is also another type of food that is perfect for breaking down stomach fat. The best thing about cabbage is that it is inexpensive to purchase and is low in carbohydrates and calories. This vegetable also contains calcium, making it an excellent choice for people who can't digest dairy products and need to increase the amount of calcium that they ingest.

Cantaloupe

Cantaloupe is also referred to as a muskmelon in certain parts of the world. This fruit is high in Vitamin A and in Vitamin C.

Cantaloupe is a good source of fiber which means that you will feel full after eating the fruit. This can help to reduce the amount of calories that you ingest. Fiber also helps to keep your digestive tract clean and it can help to stabilize your blood sugar levels and increase your metabolism.

Carrots

Carrots are another negative calorie food. You will actually spend more calories digesting the food than you ingested when you ate them. This is because carrots are relatively difficult for your body to break down and digest.

For this reason, carrots are the perfect snack to eat when you want to eat something crunchy. Eating carrots will also fill you up. Because of this, you may want to eat some carrots before you sit down to eat a meal. You may be pleasantly surprised to find that eating carrots can help you to lose weight.

Cauliflower

Cauliflower is an incredible vegetable. In fact, mashed cauliflower can be used instead of mashed potatoes if you are on a low carbohydrate diet.

Besides that, the vegetable contains no fat and is high in Vitamin C. Vitamin C can help to boost the immune system as well as to flush out fat from the body.

Finally, if you are hungry or want a crunchy snack, try munching on cauliflower instead of eating potato chips or other high calorie crunchy foods.

If you are looking to spice up your cauliflower snack, dip each piece in some hummus before eating.

Celery

Celery is an incredible vegetable. While most people eat the vegetable with peanut butter or chopped up in salads and other foods, it can be eaten by itself as a great snack.

Not many people know that celery is full of calcium. Calcium is good for your bones, but it can also help to jump start your endocrine system. This can also help to break down the fat that has accumulated in your body.

Celery is also considered to be a natural diuretic. This means that eating celery can help to flush your system and clear out any toxins.

Of course, if you are looking for a crunchy afternoon snack, celery is the perfect thing for you! If you want to keep your calorie consumption to a minimum, it is probably best to avoid dipping the celery in some high fat dressing before you eat it.

Cherries

Cherries are contain vitamins and antioxidants. Recent studies show that one of the antioxidants contained in cherries is effective at reducing belly fat.

Cherries are also low in fat and have a high water content. This means that they They have tons of nutritional benefits – vitamins, antioxidants and other compounds to keep the body healthy.

Some studies that have been done on the pigment contained in the cherries shows that the pigment can help to reduce pain, and inflammation. If you have arthritis, you may want to try this natural remedy to see if you find relief. The pigment has also been shown to help reduce cholesterol when cherries are eaten daily.

Cherries also have high potassium levels. Potassium helps to regulate your body's ability to retain water and to flush out toxins.

Chives

Chives are a member of the onion and leek family, and are full of nutrients.

But just like onions, they stimulate weight loss due to their richness in chromium.

Chromium is a nutrient that that improves the efficiency of insulin in the blood stream. If you have improper insulin levels in your bloodstream, you will feel sluggish and hungry. Some people create further problems by snacking on sugar laden foods or foods that are full of starch. While this may give them a quick boost of energy, it will also lead to a crash after the sugar and carbohydrates are processed.

One way to get off the sugar cycle is to make sure you have enough chromium in your body to keep you full of energy so that you can burn off excess fat.

The best part about chives is that they are easy to grow at home. They also complement almost any meal perfectly.

Cod

Cod is a type of fish that is packed with protein. Because of this, it is a great choice when you are looking for a fat burning food.

This fish is also rich in Omega 3-fatty acids which help to speed up your metabolism rates. Omgea-3 fatty acids also help to control the levels of leptin available in your body. This hormone also helps to increase metabolism.

If you do not like fish, you can try taking fish oil in capsules. However, it is best to get your nutrition from your food whenever possible instead of using supplements.

Corn

Corn is a popular summer time vegetable. This vegetable is very high in fiber and can help to flush waste out of your body. Corn is also very good to eat during a meal to decrease the amount of calories you ingest during your meal.

Cranberries

For centuries, women have eaten cranberries to help prevent urinary tract infections. In fact, the Romans were the first to extol the virtues of the cranberry.

Cranberries are low in sugar unless they have been artificially sweetened. Because of this, cranberries are great to eat as a part of a low carbohydrate diet.

Fresh cranberries can help to lower your cholesterol levels and may have other medicinal purposes too. In fact, cranberries can help your digestive tract to function properly.

Some doctors feel that cranberries are essential for your diet if you want to lose weight. This is because the fruit can help to flush toxins out of your system as well as excess water. Cranberries can also decrease the amount of fat in your body and improve your skin tone.

Cucumbers

Cucumbers are a true fat-burner because they are a great diuretic.

This means they will encourage the removal of fluids from your body.

So this will accelerate your metabolism, and expel with the waste fluids, quite a number of fat cells.

Diuretics can also break down large fatty deposits so they can be flushed out of the body.

They also have a high silicon and sulphur content which stimulate the kidneys to flush out the uric acid in the body.

The kidneys siphon off waste products from the body and will break down the fat and expel small fat particles from these waste products out of the body through excreted fluids. This adds to your health and slimming!

Chicken

Chicken or turkey is a very popular meat source for dieters. This is because chicken is full of lean protein. In addition, chicken is a thermogenic food. This is because it takes quite a bit of calories just to digest the food.

Chicken can help to keep you feeling full a long time after the meal. This can help to control your appetite.

Chillies

Chillies are a super food when it comes to burning calories. According to research, you can burn calories at a faster rate for up to three hours after eating chillies.

This is because chillies contain an enzyme called capsaicin. This enzyme increases your metabolism and enables you to burn fat at a faster rate.

Chickpeas

Chickpeas are also called garbanzo beans. These beans are a complete protein source. They are also low in fat and contain a number of important nutrients.

The peas are full of fiber. Because of this, they can help to lower cholesterol levels as well as blood sugar levels.

If you like chickpeas, you may also want to try using chickpea flour in your recipes. Using this type of flour is especially popular if you are on a gluten free or wheat free diet.

"D"

Daikon Radish

Although you may not have heard of this type of radish, you may have eaten it along with your sushi. This vegetable is low in calories and is a great choice for a snack if you want to lose weight.

It is also high in 3 enzymes called diastase, amylase, and esterase. These enzymes help to digest fatty foods and foods high in starch.

Some studies have shown that this particular type of radish may actually help in preventing cancer too.

Damsum Plum

Plums are loaded with Vitamin A, Vitamin B and Vitamin C. Plums also have a generous quantity of potassium and fiber.

Together, these vitamins and minerals help to keep your heart functioning at maximum efficiency. Plums will also help your immune system too because they contain phenols which are a type of antioxidant.

Plums are also considered to be a negative calorie food because your can burn more calories digesting the food than you will gain by ingesting it.

Dandelion Greens

The roots and the leaves of the dandelion plant have been used for centuries to treat numerous ailments. This is ironic because most people today regard the plant as nothing more than a lawn weed!

The leaves, which are called "greens" can be eaten as a salad. Others like to boil the leaves and eat them cooked. The leaves help to keep the liver and the kidneys functioning properly. They do act as a laxative, so it is best to not eat too many greens at once!

Dandelion tea can also be used to get rid of excess bloating or water weight. To do this, boil the leaves in water. Let the water cool and then drink.

Some people pulverize the leaves and drink the juice which is produced. The leaves are high in vitamin A as well as in vitamin C.

"E"

Eggplant

Eggplant is low in fat, sodium, and cholesterol. It has high levels of fiber, potassium and vitamins like C and K. Eggplant is also high in vitamin B as well as other minerals.

Eggplant also contains antioxidants which can help your body fight certain diseases. This vegetable is great to eat if you want to lose weight since it is high in fiber and will make you feel full. However, be sure to avoid breading the vegetable as this will add fat and calories.

Some cooks substitute eggplant in dishes that call for steak or chicken. Not only is this healthy but it also is good for your grocery budget too.

"F"

Fish

Fish is a good source of protein as well as Omega 3 fatty acids. Eating fish can help to decrease you risk of heart disease and increase your metabolism.

Some people find that eating fish actually can help them to lose weight. Experts recommend that people who have hit a plateau in their weight goals should try replacing some of the grains and meat that they eat and with fish.

Sole, Flounder and Haddock are all high in protein and low in fat. Flounder is the best fish to eat if you are looking for a protein source that is low in fat and calories. Of course, you should resist the urge to bread or fry your fish. Doing so increases the calories and the fat content of the fish.

Flax Seed Oil

Flax Seed Oil is a good source of Omega 3 and Omega 6 fatty acids. This two fatty acids are called essential fatty acids and help to increase your metabolic rate which means that you can burn more calories.

In addition, flax seed oil can help to make you feel full sooner which means you will eat less calories.

Flax seed oil has also been shown to improve mood and energy levels which can also help you to lose weight.

Remember that flax seed oil should be used primarily as a dressing or as an ingredient in a dip. Cooking flax seed oil will break down the oils and can affect the taste too.

"G"

Garlic

Garlic is one of nature's miracle foods. Garlic oil helps to reduce fat in the cells. It doesn't matter whether you eat garlic regularly or whether you take garlic capsules, the effect is the same. Doing this can help to flush fat, and toxins that have been stored in the fat from your body.

Garlic also can help to keep your blood sugar levels stable. This will prevent keep your energy levels up and help to keep your metabolism working properly. Together, this means that you will burn more body fat.

A little known fact about garlic is that it is also a natural form of antibiotic. Garlic can actually destroy a bacterial infection. You may try putting garlic tablets on a skin infection or a tooth infection to help your body heal.

Grapefruit

Grapefruit is a popular breakfast food. According to research, there is good reason to eat the fruit, even if it is at breakfast time. Grapefruit has a positive effect on the insulin levels' in your body and can also help to flush fat from your body. According to the study, grapefruit should be eaten before a meal for the best results.

However, eating grapefruit for a snack in between meals has been shown to keep insulin levels stable. Eating grapefruit between meals will reduce your hunger and encourage your body to flush fat cells.

Grapes

Grapes are low in calories. In fat, an entire cup of grapes only has about 60 calories. Grapes are also naturally sweet and can help to curb your cravings for dessert and other sweets.

Try eating some grapes when you are craving cookies, cake, or other sweets. You will get the sweetness that you crave without the calories or fat.

Green beans

Green beans are low in calories plus they are high in fiber. This means that you will feel full on less calories.

Green beans are full of minerals and vitamins. The vitamins and minerals contained in the vegetable will help to improve kidney and liver function.

Most importantly, green beans contain Vitamin C. Not only does this vitamin help your immune system, but it can also help to reduce your weight. Some studies show that eating foods with Vitamin C encourages your body to use fat for energy. When you reduce your levels of fat in your body, you will lose weight.

Green beans also contain iron. A low iron count can cause tiredness as well as decrease the ability of the immune system to fight viruses.

"H"

Honeydew melon

Honeydew melon is very sweet. This food is also high in fiber. This combination means that you can satisfy your sweet tooth and feel full without eating a lot of calories.

The best part is that this fruit is low in fat and cholesterol. Like other melons, it has a high water content and can help to keep you hydrated on a hot day.

"J"

Juniper berries

Eating juniper berries is not common, but you may want to consider adding them to your diet.

In some areas, juniper berries are used to treat different diseases because of their properties. The berries can be used as a way to decrease inflamation or to heal infections.

Juniper berries can help the urinary tract to function properly and can also help to regulate your blood pressure.

The berries are good for losing weight because they help to eliminate water retention and improve digestion.

"K"

Kale

Kale is very similar to other vegetables like broccoli and brussel sprouts. It is a great source of vitamins, minerals, and calcium. Kale also contains phyto-nutrients which help to flush toxins from the body.

This vegetable in high in fiber which will help digestive health and keep you feeling full.

"L"

Leeks

Leeks are like onions in that they help to stabilize blood sugar. Blood sugar levels that stay level mean you will have more energy and less cravings for sugary foods.

Leeks are popular in France primarily because they are a great addition to soup and other tasty dishes. Leeks are also low in calories. A cup of leeks contains only 50 calories!

Lettuce

Lettuce is another fat burning food. Lettuce is actually one of those foods that takes more calories to burn than you ingest while eating. This is called a thermogenic food. Lettuce is very low in calories. In fact, a cup of lettuce has 10 calories.

The amount of fat burning power in lettuce varies depending upon the type. The dark lettuce has more fat burning properties than do the light colored lettuce.

Lemons

Lemons have been used to fight fat for centuries. It has long been known that lemon juice can effectively flush fat from your system and break down fatty deposits in the body.

You may want to try adding some lemon to your water. Not only does it make the water taste great, but it also can help to remove toxins from your body. By flushing out the toxins, you may find that you are able to shed those unwanted pounds.

Lemons can also help to reduce cholesterol levels as they increase the effectiveness of the liver and pancreas.

The best part is that adding lemons to your diet is very easy. Just squeeze a lemon over your fish or chicken during meals. Lemons can also be used to flavor salads as well as water.

Limes

Limes are full of Vitamin C which can help to manufacture a chemical called carnitine. Carnitine helps to metabolize or flush out fat from your system.

In addition, limes are a negative calorie food as it actually takes more calories to digest the lime than the lime provides when eaten.

You can squeeze limes on your seafood or into your water. If you are watching calories, you may want to think twice before drinking beer, even if you add lime juice.

Lobster

Lobster is a great source of protein. In addition, it is low in fat unless it is eaten with butter. Lobster is also high in Omega 3 fatty acids.

One little known fact about lobster is that it is a negative calorie food. In other words, you will use up more calories digesting lobster than you will by eating the lobster.

To get the biggest benefit from lobster, you should refrain from slathering butter on the meat. This will effectively add lots of calories, fat, and cholesterol to an otherwise healthy food.

Lentils

Lentils are a great food for dieters. These beans are low in fat and calories. They contain a lot of protein as well as iron.

Lentils also are high in fiber which helps to keep you full and regulate your blood sugar levels.

Probably the best part about lentils is that they are inexpensive to purchase. You can use lentils in soup, pasta, and salad.

"M"

Mushrooms

Mushrooms are a great vegetable to eat either raw or cooked. Cooked mushrooms have long been used by vegetarians as a meat substitute.

Cooked mushrooms are also higher in nutrients than raw mushrooms. For this reason, you may want to consider cooking them.

Mushrooms are full of fiber and can help to fill you up. Mushrooms are also low in fat. However, make sure that you don't add fat to your diet by cooking them in butter or dipping them in vegetable dip.

Remember that you should purchase your mushrooms from a store or other reputable source. Gathering your own mushrooms can be dangerous, especially if you do not know how to distinguish between poisonous varieties and edible varieties.

Mango

Mangos are low in calories and filled with fiber. This combination makes them the perfect dieting food.

Mango is another negative calorie food in that it takes more calories to digest the food than it does to eat it.

Despite the fact that the mango is healthy, it has a bad reputation. This is because mango is often featured in high calorie treats, drinks, and confections.

Mango will not cause you to gain weight. However, if you eat mango cake or drink mango shakes, you probably will gain weight due to the extra calories in these treats.

Besides all of this, mangos also contain a lot of beta-carotene.

Meat

Believe it or not, eating meat can also help to boost your metabolism so that you can lose weight. For the best results, you will want to eat lean beef.

Eating protein every day will help you to keep your lean body mass which will help to keep your metabolism high. If your metabolism is high, you will burn the maximum amount of calories possible as well as using up fat deposits.

Lean meat is also a good source of vitamins and iron. Some cuts of meat like sirloin have a 2 to 1 ratio of protein to fat.

According to studies,not all saturated fat is bad. In fact, you need some to maintain energy. However, if you have been eating a lot of fat in your diet, you may want to watch the amount of fat you ingest.

Meat from grass fed cattle is healthier than grain fed cattle. This is because the pasture fed animals have less amounts of fat. If you can choose which type of meat, this is the best type to eat.

"N"

Nectarine

Nectarines are a great choice for a snack. This fruit actually has protein, but is still low in calories and fat. Of course, it is high in fiber and full of nutrients like other fruits.

Nectarines are actually a type of citrus fruit, although they look like peaches without the fuzz. A nectarine contains a high amount of vitamin C. In addition, a cup of the fruit only contains 80 calories!

Besides all these good attributes, nectarines also contain minerals like potassium and calcium. Together, these minerals help to flush out excess fluid and ensure proper hydration.

"O"

Oatmeal

Oatmeal can help you to lose weight an lower your cholesterol. This is because oatmeal is high in fiber which helps you to feel full after eating. The fiber also regulates digestion and stabilizes blood sugar levels. This means that you are less likely to crave sugary snacks.

If you pair oatmeal with protein, you will feel full longer and you will have more energy.

Oatmeal can be sweetened with natural sweetners or eaten with berries. If you still do not like the taste of oatmeal, you may want to make oatmeal bread or muffins. If you do this, use a low sugar and low fat recipe.

.

Okra

People have known about the healthy benefits of eating okra for centuries. This particular vegetable is high in fiber and contains a substance called mucilage. This is a glue like substance produced by plants.

Not only does mucilage help to keep your blood sugar levels stable, but it also helps to flush excess cholesterol from your body. Of course, this fiber also helps to keep your digestive system functioning properly.

Many people eat fried okra. However, eating okra this way will not give you the health benefits associated with the vegetable. For best results, try eating your okra in a stew or soup.

Orange

Most everyone knows that oranges are full of vitamin C. Not everyone knows that vitamin C is a great fat burning vitamin however.

In addition, oranges are full of fiber and can help to improve your immune system.

Some people think that real orange juice is just as good as eating an orange. This is not true. When you eat an orange, you are also eating the pulp of the fruit which contains the fiber. It is the fiber that keeps you feeling full long after you have eaten the orange. You won't get the same effect by just drinking orange juice.

Onion

Onions are a good food that have a bad reputation for causing smelly breath. The truth is that onions can help to break up fat deposits and the onions can help to increase your metabolism.
Onions can be used in salad, soups, and sandwiches. They are a very versatile vegetable.

Remember that leeks are a type of onion. Whether you choose to eat leeks or onions will depend upon your personal taste. However, the effects of eating either of the two will be the same.

"P"

Papaya

Papaya has no fat or cholesterol and is low in calories. The fruit also contains vitamin A, Vitamin C and potassium.

Besides these nutrients, papaya contains calcium and iron. Papaya fruit also have an enzyme called peptin. Peptin is known to help breakdown fat deposits in the body.

Papaya has a high fiber content which can help regulate sugar levels in the blood. Fiber also helps to keep the digestive system functioning properly.

Recent studies have shown that papaya can also be used to reduce cellulite and prevent the appearance of wrinkles when smoothed on the skin.

Peppers

Peppers contain vitamins, minerals, and a variety of other helpful nutrients.

Peppers are also a negative calorie food. It actually takes more calories to digest a pepper than you ingest when you eat a pepper. This is true regardless of the type of pepper that you eat.

Cayenne pepper has been shown to stop the body from absorbing fat. However, cayenne pepper is too hot to eat in any large quantity. Sprinkling the pepper on your food can help however.

Hot peppers are hot because of a chemical called capsaicin. This chemical has been shown in studies to lower cholesterol amounts as well as the amount of stored fat in your body.

Even sweet peppers contain chemicals that help to burn extra calories so that you lose weight.

Parsley

Usually, people think of parsley as just a nice looking garnishment on the side of a dish. Parsley isn't just a pretty looking herb!

Actually, parsley is packed with vitamins and minerals. The combination of all this makes this herb a fat fighting machine.

Parsley has been shown to stimulate bile production which can help to break down any fat that you eat.

Surprisingly, parsley also contains protein. This can help to increase your metabolism and break down fat stored in your body.

If you don't like the idea of eating parsley whole, you may try sprinkling ground parsley on your eggs or in your soup.

Finally, remember that parsley is a natural breath freshener. If you eat onions or garlic, chewing on a sprig of parsley can help to neutralize any odors.

Peaches

Peaches are loaded with vitamins, minerals and fiber. The best part is that peaches are low in calories. Each peach contains about 60 calories.

However, peaches are also packed with sugar. Because of this, it is probably best to eat them in moderation.

Pears

Pears are loaded with fiber. This fiber helps to keep your stomach feeling full and is also helpful to your digestive system. As with other fiber filled foods, pears can help to level out your blood sugar levels too.

Peas

Peas are full of fibre. In addition, they also contain protein! Peas are not a source of complete protein unless they are combined with another food source like brown rice.

Of course, fresh peas are higher in nutrients than canned peas. If you can not have fresh peas, frozen peas are the next best thing to fresh.

Pineapple

One slice of pineapple contains only about 40 calories. Pineapples also contain a large amount of water.

The fruit contains an enzyme which also helps to break down cellulite.

According to recent research, eating a slice of pineapple after a meal can help to improve digestion and lower stomach bloating.

Prunes

Just about everyone knows that prunes help digestion. Some people also have found that eating prunes can help to relieve or prevent constipation. This is due to the high amount of fiber contained in a prune.

Eating prunes isn't just helpful for your digestive system however. All that fiber can help to break down fat stores in your body too.

Pumpkin

Pumpkin is loaded with fiber, vitamins and water. Because of this, pumpkin can help you to feel full on less calories.

Pumpkin seeds are also a delicious and healthy snack. The seeds contain amino acids and minerals. The seeds also contain fiber. You can cook your own pumpkin seeds or purchase them in retail stores.

Pine-nuts

Pine nuts have a lower fat content than other fats. They also contain protein. Of course, protein helps the body to burn fat and reduce cholesterol levels.

If you are looking for a replacement for animal proteins, you may want to try pine-nuts.

"Q"

Quince

Quince is known in the Middle East because it can be used as an anti-biotic. In the Western world, people are more likely to eat quince in a jelly.

Quince is also low in fat, cholesterol and sodium. Because it is high in Vitamin C and fiber, it great for fat fighting.

"R"

Radish

There are many different types of radishes. The most popular kind are the red and white variety. This type of radish is also full of minerals.

Some radishes are negative calorie foods because it takes more to digest the vegetable than is taken in after eating it. The term for this is thermogenic.

Some people eat radishes for a snack. Most people slice them and eat them on salads. However you eat radishes, you can rest assured that they will help to keep your metabolism functioning properly.

Raspberries

Raspberries are a wonderful fat fighting food. The berries contain a large amount of fiber which slows the rate which carbohydrates are absorbed by the body. Because of this, raspberries help to control your blood sugar levels.

Raspberries also have pectic. This enzyme controls how much fat can be absorbed by cells. It also forces cells to get rid of fatty deposits. This helps to aid weight loss.

By eating raspberries, you can give your metabolism a boost and help your body to burn fat at the same time.

Red cabbage

Red cabbage can be eaten cooked or raw. Many people eat it shredded in their salads. Not only does it look attractive, but it tastes good tool.

Raw cabbage is great to eat when you want to eat something crunchy, but don't want to ingest a lot of calories. If you don't the taste of raw cabbage, you may want to try sprinkling it with some vinegar.

This vegetable also contains vitamin C, minerals, and fiber.

"S"

Spinach

Popeye and your mother were right. Spinach is good for you.

Spinach is high in vitamin A and iron and low in fat as well as calories.

When eaten regularly, spinach will help to boost your metabolism. It will also help your liver to function at peak efficiency.

If you do not like the taste of cooked spinach, you can try eating it raw in your salads.

Squash

Squash is another fiber filled vegetable. There are many different types of squash, but all of them are fiber filled.

Some people eat certain types of squash instead of foods high in carbs which others use squash as a meat substitute.

Whatever you do, do not bread and fry the squash.

This will do more harm than good. Boiling or steaming squash is a good way to eat the vegetable. You can also eat sliced squash raw in a salad.

Strawberries

Strawberries are another popular berry. This fruit contains a fat burning enzyme called adiponectin.

Strawberries also contain another enzyme called leptin which helps to increase metabolism and decrease food cravings.

By eating strawberries, you can help control the sugar levels in your blood. In turn, this will reduce cravings for sugary foods.

However, you can't slather the berries in cream and sugar if you want to experience the benefits of eating strawberries. Instead, cut them up and eat them with yogurt or with your cereal.

String beans

String beans are a popular summer vegetable that are grown in many gardens across the country. String beans are also found in the frozen food aisle or in the canned vegetable aisle of the grocery store.

For the most nutrients, use fresh string beans from the garden or fresh beans purchase at a local market.

Eating this vegetable can help fill you up and flush toxins from your body. This combination will help you to lose weight and increase your metabolism.

Scallions or Spring Onions

Scallions are a type of onion. These vegetables are good for regulating blood sugar and decreasing your appetite.

Scallions are great to eat in soups or sprinkled over various dishes.

Spices

Spicy food is also good for increasing your metabolism. Foods like red peppers, cayenne pepper and hot sauce will all increase your metabolism and help you to burn more calories.

You don't have to eat excessively hot food in order to boost your metabolism. You can do so by putting crushed red peppers, or chilies on your food. You can also sprinkle cayenne pepper on your food.

"T"

Tomato

It doesn't matter whether you consider the tomato a fruit or a vegetable, this food still contains a lot of vitamins and anti-oxidants.

Tomatoes also have a chemical called carnitine which helps to break down your body fat. Unlike other foods that lose their nutrients when cooked, a tomato actually releases more carnitine when cooked.

You can eat tomatoes raw or eat them after they have been cooked. Either way, you will still be getting all the benefits that this food has to offer.

Tangerine

Tangerines are low in calories. In fact, a large tangerine has only about 43 of them.

Tangerines also have large amounts of Vitamin C which can help improve your metabolism. Tangerines are sweet too. The next time you want to eat something sweet, you may try eating a tangerine instead of a cookie.

Turnips

A cup of turnips contains about 36 calories. Because of this, turnips are popular with dieters. Turnips are also considered to be a negative calorie food.

You may want to use turnips as a potato substitute to save calories or to help increase your metabolism.

"U"

Ugli

The ugli is a fruit grown only in Jamaica. It can be found sporadically in other areas. If you have never been to Jamaica, you may not know what the ugli is. The ugli has been described as a cross between a lemon, lime and nectarine.

The fruit contains an enzyme that can help absorb fat in the body and level the sugar in the blood stream.

Ugli fruit are also full of Vitamin C and pectic. This combination also helps to increase the fat burning power of this fruit.

"V"

Venison

Venison is an iron rich meat that contains plenty of protein. It tastes great in stews, soups, and other types of dishes.

Iron is important and can help you to achieve your weight loss goals. Foods that are rich in iron carry oxygen to the blood. These cells then provide energy for muscles during exercise.

Vinegar

Apple cider vinegar has been used by people to lose weight for years. According to experts, the nutrients and enzymes in the vinegar help to reduce a person's appetite while increasing metabolism.

This type of vinegar also removes toxins from your blood stream, levels out your blood sugar levels, and helps to balance the acid in your body.

One of the best ways to incorporate apple cider vinegar into your diet is to use it as a salad dressing. You can add it by itself or mix it with olive oil.

"W"

Watermelon

Watermelon is also full of fiber. This incredible fruit is also considered to be a negative calorie food.

Not only is the food cool and refreshing, but it also helps to increase your metabolism in the process.

Today, watermelon has gotten a bad reputation. This is primarily because watermelon flavor is used in many high calorie treats. The truth is that watermelon is not high in calories at all.

Watermelon only contains natural sugars and it is very high in water content. This high water content can help to flush fat from your system.

If you are trying to lose weight, but want to eat constantly, you may want to try to eat watermelon when you are hungry. This is because it is low in calories and actually burns more calories to digest than it adds when eaten.

"X"

Xiuga

The xiuga is a type of Asian watermelon. The xiuga is similar to a watermelon except it is smaller in size.

"Y"

Yam

Yams are also known as sweet potatoes. This is probably because yams are very sweet.

While the yam is sweet, it does not overload the blood stream with sugar. This vegetable actually helps to control blood sugar.

In addition, yams also contain a number of vitamins and minerals.

However, all of these good things can be undone. Many people eat sweet potatoes in pie or topped with sugar, cinnamon, or marshmallows. Remember that you won't lose fat and increase your metabolism when you slather good food with high calorie and high sugar foods.

For the best outcome, enjoy sweet potatoes or yams by themselves.

"Z"

Zucchini

Otherwise known as Courgettes, these are low in fat, high in water content and a good source of folic acid, fibre and potassium.

You will feel fuller for longer with less calories.

Conclusion

The above list should go a long way to helping you choose fat fighting foods. Over time, these foods should help you to lose weight and stay healthy. Of course, you will also be able to avoid feeling hungry in the process.

For best results, start of slowly incorporating foods into your diet. Don't feel that you need to change your diet drastically overnight.

Remember that your body burns calories when processing the foods that you eat. If you reduce your calorie consumption too much, your body will respond by lowering your metabolic rate and burning less calories.

In order to prevent this from happening, you should eat small but frequent "meals" through out the day. This will prevent your metabolism from reducing and will help to increase your weight loss.

As you have seen, some of the foods listed here will help to increase your metabolism and provide nutrients without providing a lot of calories in the process.

If you are hungry for sweets, try snacking on one of the sweet fruits listed above. You will ingest less calories and you won't have to deal with the consequences of digesting processed sugar.

If you want to learn more about healthy eating, you may want to try reading my book entitled *Healthy Eating.*

I wish you the best as you begin your journey to eat better and burn more fat.

C Elias

21883125R00038

Made in the USA
Lexington, KY
04 April 2013